Essential Oils for Hair

Get Healthy, Beautiful and Full of Body Hair Today by Applying These Simple to use Essential Oil Tricks for Your Hair and Scalp!

Recipes Included!

Table of Contents:

Introduction

I want to thank you and congratulate you for downloading the book, *"Essential Oils for Hair: Get Healthy, Beautiful and Full of Body Hair Today by Applying these Simple to use Essential Oil Tricks for Your Hair and Scalp! Recipes Included!*

This book contains proven steps and strategies on how to take care of your hair and scalp using essential oils. You will also learn how to make your own hair care products using essential oils; that way, you're sure about what goes to your hair and that the results are suitable to your hair type.

Making our hair and scalp clean is part of our personal hygiene. However, most of the products available in the market have chemicals that can damage our hair and scalp. One way to avoid damaging our hair and scalp is to make sure that we are using hair products that are chemical-free. Consequently, the best way to ensure that the products we use are all natural and chemical-free is if we made it on our own.

Essential oils are one of the main ingredients for making our hair clean and healthy. This book will teach you how to use different essential oils to make your own natural hair products and achieve a beautiful, full body and shiny hair.

Thanks again for downloading this book. I hope you enjoy it!

responsibility of the recipient reader. Under no circumstances will any legal responsibility or blame be held against the publisher for any reparation, damages, or monetary loss due to the information herein, either directly or indirectly.

Respective authors own all copyrights not held by the publisher.

The information herein is offered for informational purposes solely, and is universal as so. The presentation of the information is without contract or any type of guarantee assurance.

The trademarks that are used are without any consent, and the publication of the trademark is without permission or backing by the trademark owner. All trademarks and brands within this book are for clarifying purposes only and are the owned by the owners themselves, not affiliated with this document.

Chapter 1: What Essential Oils Can Do For Your Hair

Hair that is beautiful, shining and full of body can enhance the natural beauty and self- confidence of a person.

But more than something that looks nice, your hair also protects the body, especially the head. It protects the head from the cold and heat. It also traps dirt and harmful substances that may harm the scalp. Hence, it is important that the hair should be kept clean and healthy.

However, everyday grooming can cause damage to the hair. Even those practices that are essential to our hair and scalp hygiene can be harmful if done incorrectly or done over a long time.

Here are some of the practices that can be both essential and damaging to the hair.

1. Frequent Brushing.

Some people suggest that brushing the hair for at least 1000 times a day could stimulate beautiful growth and shine. Hair experts, however, say that the truth about this practice depends on the kind of hair.

Brushing normal hair frequently may not be harmful. Frequent brushing dry and brittle hair can cause split-ends or hair fall. Brushing oily hair frequently can make it oilier and more susceptible to dirt.

2. Using Shampoo and conditioners every day.

Shampoo is used to clean the hair, whereas conditioner is used to make the hair smooth and manageable. Most shampoos and conditioners have chemicals that weaken the hair and the scalp after a while of using.

Hair experts say that some shampoo can wash off the natural oil that the body feeds the hair. On the other hand, the conditioners make the hair become dependent on the synthetic oil that the conditioners provide. Instead of making the hair healthy, these products may make the hair vulnerable.

3. Using commercial hair mousse, hair sprays and leave-on conditioners.

Hair mousse, hair sprays and leave-on conditioners help in keeping the hair manageable during styling. Though natural essential oils are added to these products, manufacturers are using synthetic chemicals to preserve the oils. The synthetic chemicals may make the hair unhealthy and difficult to manage after a long time of using it.

Essential Oils for Hair

Because of the aforementioned practices, it is necessary that the hair is supplemented with natural vitamins and minerals to maintain its health, body and beauty. These natural vitamins and minerals may be acquired by using or applying essential oils directly to the scalp and hair.

There are many kinds of essential oils that can be used on the hair. Each essential oil has different effects on the hair.

Below is a chart that shows the basic essential oils and what type of hair or scalp it is recommended to be applied to.

Essential Oil	Type of Hair
Avocado Olive Castor Sweet Almond Coconut Grapefruit Aloe Vera Sunflower Seed Sesame Oil	Thinning Hair or Hair that is Prone to Hair fall
Coconut Shea butter Castor Jojoba Olive Sunflower Seed	Dry and Brittle Hair Dry, itchy scalp Frizzy, dry curly hair

Coconut Jojoba Sunflower	Normal Hair
Jojoba Aloe Vera Avocado Coconut Castor Sesame Grapefruit	Oily hair Scalp with Dandruff

Chapter 2: The Wonders of the Three Basic Essential Oils for Hair

The three basic essential oils for hair, as seen in the chart in the first chapter, are Jojoba Oil, Sunflower Oil, and Coconut oil. These three oils are usually used as bases for other essential oils and natural hair products. These essential oils are also called carrier oils.

Jojoba Oil

Jojoba oil is an extract from Jojoba seeds. It comes from a shrub that is abundant in Arizona and California.

Jojoba oil is a known natural ingredient in many cosmetic products.

What it does to the hair

When applied, jojoba oil moisturizes the hair strands. It also nourishes the scalp. According to some studies, jojoba oil is not actually an oil but a wax. It is similar to the serum produced by the oil glands in the body. When applied to the scalp or skin, it makes the body regulate the production of serum. This makes the body produce just enough oil to make the hair and the scalp healthy, shiny and beautiful.

Coconut Oil

Coconut oil is an extract from the meat of the mature coconut. It is extracted from the coconut by two processes.

The dry process involves drying the coconut meat and then mashing it together with some solvent. The oil derived from the dry process is clear and thin. This kind of coconut oil is often used in commercial hair products.

The wet process involves squeezing the coconut milk from the coconut gratings. The coconut milk is boiled until the coconut oil separates from the solids. The oil derived from the wet process is brown in color and thicker. It also emits a cooked oil smell.

What it does to the hair

Applying pure coconut oil on the hair may make it smooth and shiny. Applying it directly on the scalp will strengthen the scalp and make it resistant from dandruff. The coconut oil can also be used as a home remedy for treating dandruff.

Coconut oil is also known for repairing hair breakage. Putting the oil on the ends of the hair may repair the split ends.

In cold countries, coconut oil is used as natural styling liquid because it condenses in cold temperature. Thus, it can hold the hair style.

Coconut oil is also used for treatment of lice. It helps the hair less prone to breakage when combed with a lice-remover. It also forces the lice to remain on the surface of the hair and away from the scalp. Thus, the lice are easier to remove.

Sunflower Oil

Sunflower oil is a new breakthrough in hair

products. It was not believed to be beneficial to the hair until recently. It was proven that its potassium, vitamin A, B, C and E contents can stimulate hair growth.

What it does to the hair

Aside from conditioning the hair and stimulating healthy growth, sunflower oil also protects the hair and scalp from ultraviolet lights.

It is believed that the oil has anti-fungal benefits and is effective in eliminating dandruff and scalp itchiness.

Since it is rich in vitamin E, it keeps the scalp hydrated. When the scalp is hydrated, the tendencies of itchy scalp, dandruff and lice infestations are reduced.

Chapter 3: Some Essential Oils That Can Be Used to Supplement the Carrier Oils

Carrier oils are already good for the hair on their own. But, some essential oils are added to these carrier oils to add scents or to supplement the benefits given by the carrier oils.

Below are some of these beneficial essential oils:

Aloe Vera Oil

Aloe Vera Oil can also be used as a carrier oil. However, the oil is so thick that it is uncomfortable to be used directly to the hair without rinsing. In its fresh state, the oil is trapped in the gel or the meat of the aloe vera plant.

Aloe Vera is known to stimulate hair growth. Though it tends to make the hair sticky, it hydrates the scalp and helps eliminates dandruff. It is also known to lower the risk of alopecia or hair loss. It also adds volume or body to the hair.

This oil is usually added to the coconut oil because the latter removes the stickiness that the Aloe Vera brings to the hair.

Lavender Oil

The Lavender oil is usually added to the carrier oil because of its scent. Many consumers chose hair products with lavender essences because of it relaxes the scalp and the head.

Aside from its scent and relaxing benefits, lavender oil can be added to the hair product in order to stimulate growth. The oil is also known to help remove dandruffs and alleviate scalp itchiness.

Chamomile Oil

Chamomile oil is known to be a soothing oil. It is usually used in massaging the body because of its calming effects.

Chamomile oil is added to the hair products to relax

the body and the scalp. It may not have a direct effect on making the hair shine or gaining hair volume, but it protects the hair from stress and lice.

Peppermint Oil

Peppermint oil helps stimulate blood flow to the scalp. It helps bring the nutrients to the scalp. This results in stronger hair roots. Thus, it helps in preventing hair loss or alopecia. It also prevents hair graying. It is also believed to make the natural color of the hair more vibrant.

The oil also has a cooling effect that stimulates hair growth. It also eliminates lice and other insects.

Tea Tree oil

Tea tree oil unblocks the oil glands in the scalp, making it healthier. The natural serum from these unblocked glands and the tea tree oil removes the dead skin cells. This results in a healthy scalp and shiny hair. Also, it revives the dead hair roots and helps recover from hair loss.

However, many people are allergic to tea tree oil. Though the oil may aid the hair and the scalp, it may cause scalp itchiness and irritations to others.

Carrot Oil

It may be surprising to know that carrot oil is used in cosmetic products, but this oil is proven to be good for the hair.

Carrot oil or just the carrot fruit is known to help in rejuvenating the skin because of its anti-cancer and antioxidant benefits. As it rejuvenates the body, it also revives the scalp and the hair follicles. It helps prevent alopecia and also helps stimulate hair regrowth.

Rosemary Oil

Some studies show that rosemary oil is not just a

fragrance oil for cosmetics but a helpful oil. It helps moisturize the hair follicles. It hydrates the scalp and helps eliminate dandruffs. It also stimulates healthy hair growth.

Many hair experts recommend using hair products with rosemary oil for women who want to have strong and healthy long hairs.

Lemon or Citric Oils

Lemon or citric oils are essential oils that are mainly used because of their scent. But, more than its scent, lemon is known to help revitalize the scalp and hair. Some studies also show that lemon oil makes the natural hair color become more vibrant.

Olive Oil

Olive oil can also be used as a carrier oil, but only for specific hair types. Because of its inability to condense, it is not advisable to oily and normal hair.

It may make the hair sticky and oilier. It is recommended to be used for color-treated hair. It does not strip away the hair dyes unlike jojoba and coconut oil.

Olive oil is believed to aid hair regrowth. It also strengthens the strands and makes the follicle thicker. It is also proven to help repair split ends.

Grapefruit oil

One of the breakthrough essential oils for hair is the grapefruit oil. It can be used directly on the hair or mixed with a carrier oil. It is a good hair deodorizer. It is a great hair cleanser after a swim in the sea or the pool. It cleanses the hair of salt and chlorine.

When applied to the scalp, it helps remove dandruff and stimulates hair growth.

Shea Butter

This oil comes from the Shea tree which is abundant

in Africa. The oil is high in triglycerides that it is often in the solid state. The high amount of triglycerides in Shea butter makes it a good ingredient for natural cosmetic products.

It is great for the hair because it seeps inside the scalp and the follicles when melted. The oil that did not successfully penetrate the scalp and the follicles becomes condensed and coats the hair. Thus, it makes the hair healthy inside and beautiful and shiny on the outside.

Sesame Oil (Untoasted)

The sesame oil used in hair and cosmetic products is from untoasted sesame seeds. It is a popular ingredient for hair regrowth and anti-graying hair products. The oil is proven to help minimize hair thinning or alopecia.

Sesame oil is rich in vitamin B. The vitamin is known to prevent graying of hair.

Castor Oil

Castor oil is sometimes used as substitute carrier oil for coconut oil. It helps strengthen the hair strands and stimulate faster hair growth. It also makes the hair shiny. It is highly recommended to women who want to have long hair, which is less prone to damage.

Tips on Choosing the Right Essential Oil

Not all essential oils are safe to use for everyone. Some people may be allergic to the main ingredient of the Essential oil.

Here are some tips on how to choose the right essential oil.

1. Know Your Allergies.

When a person is allergic to a certain food or substance, he may be allergic to all the products derived from that food or substance. For example, if a person is allergic to sesame seeds, he is likely to be allergic to sesame oil. Hence, he should avoid using products with sesame oil.

2. Choose the oil base on your hair type and not by fragrance.

Many people are inclined to use essential oils that are fragrant or pleasant to their nostrils instead of what is suited to their hair type. It is important to use only the essential oils that are suitable for a certain hair type to maximize the effectiveness of the essential oil. Also, using fragrance oil that is not suitable to the hair may cause the latter to become oilier or drier.

Chapter 4   Do-it-Yourself Natural Shampoos and Conditioners

Shampoo Recipes

Coconut Milk Anti-dandruff Shampoo

Ingredients:

- 1 cup fresh coconut milk*
- 1 cup liquid Castille soap
- 20 drops of Chamomile oil
- 20 drops of rosemary oil
- 30 drops of Lavender oil
- 10 drops of Tea Tree oil**

Directions:

Combine all the ingredients in a bottle. Shake the bottle until the oil and the other liquids are incorporated.

*There are two kinds of fresh coconut milk. One is diluted and the other is concentrated. The

26

concentrated one is preferred.

Canned coconut milk can be used, but because of the preservatives, it may make the shampoo less effective. Using the fresh squeezed coconut milk is better. But, before using the fresh squeezed coconut milk, scald it first to kill the bacteria and to improve its shelf life.

**If anyone in the family is allergic to tea-tree oil, you may use another type of essential oil; you may also proportionally increase one or some of the other oils in the recipe

***These shampoo should be kept in the fridge to keep the coconut milk from spoiling.

Rosemary Peppermint Home Made Shampoo

Ingredients:

- 1 cup distilled water (if clean fresh spring water is available, use it instead)
- 1 cup liquid Castile Soap
- 25 drops of rosemary oil
- 10 drops of peppermint oil
- Eucalyptus oil (optional)

Directions:

Combine all the ingredients except for the eucalyptus oil.

When using, squeeze a generous amount in the palm. Before applying the shampoo, put a drop of eucalyptus oil in the mixture. The eucalyptus oil will emphasize the scent of the rosemary and add to the coolness of the peppermint.

Coconut-Aloe Vera Shampoo for Full Body Hair

Ingredients:

- 1 cup fresh coconut milk
- ½ cup aloe vera gel or oil
- 10 drops of lavender oil
- 10 drops of chamomile oil
- 16 to 20 plastic sachets (with zip-lock, if available)

Directions:

Mix the coconut milk and the aloe vera gel. Make sure to totally incorporate the gel. Gradually drop the oils to the mixture.

Transfer the mixture equally to the plastic sachets. Freeze the mixture until it is ready to use.

To use: Take out a sachet at least three hours before taking the shower. The mixture must be thawed before it can be used.

*The mixture will not produce any lather. The aloe

vera gel and the coconut milk are sufficient to cleanse the hair strands. Massage the shampoo on the hair well.

** Because of the aloe vera gel, the hair can become a bit waxy and sticky. Hence, it is not advisable for people with oily hair. It can help with dry and brittle hair, but the mixture will be sticky during the lathering. It is recommended to add 1 tablespoon of jojoba or sunflower oil to the mixture to make it suited for dry hair.

Lathering Aloe Vera Shampoo (For Dry Hair with Dandruff)

Ingredients:

- 1 cup liquid Castille soap
- 1 cup aloe vera gel or oil
- 4 teaspoon vegetable glycerin
- ¼ cup of sunflower oil (coconut oil or jojoba oil can be used, too)
- 20 drops of rosemary oil and/or lavender oil

Directions:

Combine the aloe vera gel or oil, glycerin and the sunflower oil. Gradually drop the other essential oils. Incorporate well.

Fold in the oils to the Castille soap. Mix slowly just to incorporate the ingredients. Keep the bubbling of the liquid soap to a minimal.

Transfer to a shampoo bottle.

*Fresh gel from the aloe vera plant can be more effective, but it will create lumps on the mixture. If using the fresh gel, push the gel through a strainer when adding it to the oil. The strainer will break the aloe vera into finer gels and make it easier to dissolve.

Avocado Anti-hair Fall Shampoo

Ingredients:

- 2 tablespoon avocado oil
- 1 ½ cup distilled or fresh spring water
- ¾ cup Castile soap
- 1 tablespoon vegetable glycerin
- 1 teaspoon carrot oil
- 1 teaspoon rosemary oil
- 1 teaspoon of grapefruit, chamomile or lemon oil

Directions:

Combine all the ingredients except for the Castile soap. Incorporate the oils and the glycerin well.

Fold the mixture to the Castile soap. Mix slowly to minimize the bubbles. Transfer the mixture in a bottle.

*Since carrot oil is difficult to find, you can use olive or sunflower oil instead

Green Tea with Honey Shampoo

Ingredients:

- ¼ cup dried herbal tea leaves (sage, thyme, peppermint, rosemary, basil)
- 1 stalk lemon grass
- 1 cup distilled water
- 1 tablespoon olive oil
- 1 teaspoon raw honey (if honey is not available, substitute with glycerin)
- 1 cup Castile soap

Directions:

Boil the water with the herbal leaves and the lemon grass. If using fresh leaves, increase the measurement of the leaves to 1 cup. Strain the liquid.

Let the liquid cool until lukewarm. Add the olive oil and honey. Mix well.

Fold the mixture to the Castile soap. The mixture can easily bubble because it contains water, so be gentle when mixing.

*This shampoo does not need additional essential oils because the herbal tea leaves are already rich in nutrients. If desired, add some fragrance oil to lessen or eliminate the herbal tea fragrance.

*This shampoo works great for color-treated hair. It also prevents hair graying.

*Brunettes who want to darken their natural brown hair should replace the tea with fresh brewed coffee. Just add 5 to 10 drops of eucalyptus oil to lessen the coffee smell.

Conditioner Recipes

Why condition first before shampooing?

Shampoos are usually water based, whereas conditioners are oil-based. If shampoo is applied prior to the conditioner, the hair follicles and the scalp would absorbed the water. Since oil has a lesser density than water, it may no longer seep into the follicle or the scalp but will remain only on the surface.

Thus, oil-based conditioners should be applied first in order to allow the oil to deeply penetrate the scalp and the follicles. Shampooing afterwards will no longer rid the hair of the nutrients from the oil.

Basic Coconut Hair Conditioner

This conditioner is suited for any hair types, but it is more effective on dry and frizzy hair. It is applied before shampooing the hair and not after. Thus, adding fragrance oil is only optional.

Ingredients:

- 1 cup coconut oil
- ½ cup Shea butter
- ¼ cup avocado oil
- 20 drops of chamomile and/or lavender drops (optional)
- 10 to 16 plastic sachets

Directions:

Since Shea butter is often in a solid state, melt it over a double boiler. Melting it in the microwave can be done too, but be careful not to cook the butter.

Add the other oils while the butter is still warm. Let the mixture cool down a little before transferring it in plastic sachets.

Place the sachets in the fridge.

To use: Thaw the mixture by soaking the sachet in hot water for 2 to 3 minutes. Wet the hair thoroughly. Apply the conditioner. Leave it on the hair for 10 to 15 minutes. Rinse with warm water. Use any of the lathering natural shampoos. Rinse thoroughly.

Tip: If the hair is thin, apply the conditioner from the middle to the ends only. If applied on the top hair, the hair may look flat and thinner.

Avocado-Honey Hair Conditioner

This conditioner is an anti-hair fall and anti-dandruff conditioner. It can also be used as a treatment for lice.

Ingredients:

- 1 cup pitted ripe avocado
- 3-4 tablespoon of honey (raw or royal honey)
- 2 tablespoon sunflower oil (coconut oil and jojoba oil can be used, too)
- ¼ cup aloe vera oil or gel
- 10 drops of lemon essence
- 1 teaspoon lemon juice

Directions:

Whip the ripe avocado until it is smooth and buttery. While whipping, add the honey, sunflower oil, aloe vera oil or gel, lemon juice and lemon essence. Incorporate the ingredients well.

Let the mixture pass thru a strainer to eliminate the

lumps. Transfer the smooth mixture in a jar or a bottle.

To use: Use a tablespoon of the mixture. Spread it evenly from scalp to the ends of the hair. Cover the hair with a shower cap for 15 minutes. For dry and frizzy hair, it is recommended to use warm or hot towels to wrap the hair instead.

After 15 minutes, rinse the hair thoroughly. Use any of the lathering natural shampoos to thoroughly cleanse the hair.

Deep Hair Conditioner for Dry and Brittle hair

Ingredients:

- 1 cup ripe banana or avocado
- 1 cup plain, sugarless yogurt
- 1 cup extra virgin coconut or olive oil
- ¼ cup honey

Directions:

Blend the banana or avocado with the extra virgin coconut or olive oil until the mixture reaches a smooth consistency. Add the yogurt and the honey. Mix in the blender for a minute. Pass the mixture in a strainer to keep it lump free. Place the mixture in the container.

To use: Apply on wet hair before shampooing. Leave the conditioner on the hair for 30 minutes for the treatment to work well. Rinse thoroughly and shampoo.

Tip: If your hair is colored treated, use only olive oil. Coconut oil may strip the color from your hair.

Repairing Hair Conditioner

Ingredients:

- 1 egg
- 1 tablespoon sunflower oil
- 1 tablespoon castor oil
- 1 cup plain, sugarless yogurt

Directions:

Using a whisk, whip the egg until frothy. In another bowl, whip the yogurt until it becomes smooth. Add the sunflower oil and the castor oil. Then add the whipped egg. Mix well.

To use: Apply the conditioner on a damp hair. Use more of the conditioners on the ends to repair the split ends. Cover with a plastic shower cap for at least an hour. Rinse thoroughly and shampoo.

Tip: If you want the conditioner to have a longer shelf-life and to be salmonella free, substitute 1 egg with ¼ cup of plain mayonnaise.

Anti-Dandruff and Anti-itch Hair Conditioner

Ingredients:

- ¼ cup sesame oil (not the toasted sesame oil used in cooking)
- 2 tablespoons Aloe Vera oil or gel
- 1 tablespoon coconut oil
- 1 cup plain, sugarless yogurt
- 10 drops of peppermint oil or tea tree oil

Directions:

Whip the yogurt until smooth. Add the oils one by one while whipping. Place the conditioner in a plastic bottle.

To use: Apply on wet hair. Apply more of the conditioner on the scalp. Cover with a shower plastic cap for an hour. Rinse thoroughly. Wash with any aloe vera shampoo for better result.

Chapter 5: Leave-on Conditioners, Hair Mousses and Other Hair Treatment Recipes

Leave-on Conditioners

Any of the carrier oils can be directly used as leave-on conditioners for the hair. Just put a teaspoon of the oil in the palm and apply onto wet or damp hair. The oil will keep the hair moisturized and manageable all day. For better scent and effectiveness, just add a few drops of peppermint, rosemary or lavender oil. The oil can work as a light hair mousse, too.

But for some who are not comfortable about using pure oil on their hair, here are some water-based leave-on conditioner recipes.

Leave-on Conditioner for Normal Hair

Ingredients:

- 1 cup water
- 1 teaspoon Lavender oil
- 1/8 cup jojoba oil
- 1/8 cup vegetable glycerin

Directions:

Combine all the ingredients. Mix well. Transfer the liquid in a spray bottle. Shake the bottle first before spraying the mixture on the hair.

Leave-on Conditioner for Dry Hair

Ingredients:

- 1 cup pure, undiluted coconut milk
- ¼ cup coconut oil
- 1 teaspoon rosemary or peppermint oil

Directions:

Combine all the ingredients. Shake well. Place in a spray bottle. Shake the bottle first before applying to the hair. For best result, spray the mixture on the scalp and spread the mixture by combing the hair.

Leave-on Conditioner for Oily Hair or Color-Treated Hair

Ingredients:

- 1 cup rose water
- 1/8 cup sunflower oil or olive oil
- 1/8 glycerin

Directions:

Combine all the ingredients. Mix well. Transfer in a spray bottle. Shake the bottle before using on hair.

Tip: In applying the conditioner, just apply it from the middle to the ends of the hair. Do not apply it on top because the hair will become oilier. The hair may also look messy or flat.

*Rosewater is already fragrant. There is no need to add fragrance oil. If preferred, a teaspoon of grapefruit oil or lavender oil can be added to the mixture to neutralize the strong scent of rose.

Hair Mouse Recipes

Hair mousse is usually used to keep curly hair manageable. It is different from leave-on conditioner because it is used for styling hair and not just to keep hair frizz-free

Coconut oil as Hair Mouse

Coconut oil is a great natural mousse. Take a teaspoon or two of the coconut oil. Place it in the fridge for three to five minutes so that the oil will become a little buttery in terms of consistency. Apply it directly on the hair. Then, blow dry.

It is necessary for the coconut oil to be buttery during the application so that it will not drip when the hair is blow dried.

Shea Butter as Hair Mousse

Shea butter can be applied to the hair directly as a hair mousse. However, unlike the coconut oil, Shea butter has a strong scent that can be uncomfortable or offensive to the nose. Adding peppermint or eucalyptus oil in the butter before the application is highly recommended. The fragrance oil will help reduce the smell of the butter.

To use Shea butter as a mouse, whip the butter until creamy. Add the essential oils and apply directly on a damp hair.

Below are some other Hair Mousse Recipes for different types of hair.

Hair Mousse for Dry Curly Hair

Ingredients:

- ½ cup olive oil
- ½ cup Shea butter
- 40 drops peppermint essential oil
- 10 drops of lavender or rosemary oil
- 10 drops of tea-tree oil

Directions:

Whip the Shea butter and half of the olive oil in a

mixing bowl until fully incorporated. Add the essential oils and mix again for at least 2 minutes. Slowly add the remaining olive oil while mixing.

Place the mixture in a container and keep in a dark and dry place.

To use: Use a teaspoon of the mixture. Add a little if the hair is past the shoulder length. Spread the mixture evenly on a damp hair. Blow the hair dry.

*This mousse is made specifically for color-treated, curly, dry hair. If the hair is not color-treated, using coconut oil is recommended. Or if preferred, the carrier oil can be half olive oil and half coconut oil. Just make sure to add the coconut oil first on the Shea butter.

*If allergic to tea-tree oil, lemon or citric oil can be used as a substitute. Eucalyptus oil can also be used as a substitute or a supplement for the peppermint.

Mango and Coconut Hair Mousse

Ingredients:

- ½ cup mango butter
- ½ cup coconut oil
- 20 drops of lemon or citric oils
- 10 drops of carrot oil or vitamin E essence

Directions:

Melt the mango butter in the double boiler. Add the coconut oil. Mix over the double boiler until the mixture reaches a creamy consistency. Remove from heat. Add the essential oils.

Place the mixture in a glass jar. Use it on a damp hair as a mouse or a styling cream.

Hair Styling Gel and Pomade Recipes

Aloe Vera as hair styling gel

Aloe Vera gel can be used directly on the hair as a styling gel. The stickiness of the aloe vera gel can hold simple styles. The only downside of using the natural gel is the strong smell of the plant. But adding fragrance oil can easily neutralize it.

To make a fresh homemade aloe vera gel, split the plant in half and scrape the meat. Place the meat in a fine strainer. Push the meat to the strainer in order to extract the gel and oil of the plant. Add some drops of lavender or peppermint essential oil.

Apply the gel directly to the hair and style as desired.

Rose-Aloc Vera Hair Styling Gel

Ingredients:

- 1 teaspoon unflavored and uncolored gelatin
- 1 cup rose water
- ½ cup fresh aloe vera gel or oil

Directions:

Dissolve the gelatin in the rose water. Bring to a quick boil over high heat. Remove from fire. Stir the water until the gelatin begins to set. Add the aloe vera gel. If preferred, add 10 drops of lavender or rosemary oil. Mix until the gelatin is coarsely set. Transfer the mixture in a plastic or glass bottle.

To use: Apply on wet or dry hair. Style the hair as desired.

*For stronger hold, increase the gelatin to two teaspoons.

All Natural Pomade

Ingredients:

- 3 tablespoons Shea Butter
- 2 tablespoons Jojoba oil or coconut oil
- 1 tablespoon arrowroot powder
- 2 tablespoons beeswax
- 10 drops of peppermint oil (optional)
- Vitamin E extract*

Directions:

Cook the beeswax and the Shea butter in a double boiler. Let it cook until the Shea butter and beeswax becomes clear.

In a small bowl, dissolve the arrowroot powder in the coconut oil. Add the essential oil, if using, and the vitamin E extract.

Add the oil mixture to the Shea butter mixture. Using an electric mixer, whip the mixture until it holds a pudding consistency. Transfer the mixture in a small container.

To use: Get a pea size of the mixture. Spread it evenly to the hair. This product is more suited for men than women.

*Vitamin E is necessary to extend the shelf life of the pomade.

Hot Oil Treatment Recipes

Carrier Oils as Hot Oil Treatment

The three carrier oils can be used for hot oil treatments for any type of hairs, except for color treated hairs.

To use them for the hot oil treatment, just heat a few tablespoons of any or combination of the carrier oils for an hour over a double boiler. Let it cool down until it is safe to touch. Apply it evenly to the hair and the scalp.

Cover the hair with a plastic shower cap for an hour. For a shorter curing period, wrap the hair with a hot towel instead for 15 to 30 minutes. An electric hair steamer can also be used for faster curing. Rinse thoroughly.

Hot Oil Treatment for Color-treated Hair

Ingredients:

- 1 tablespoon olive oil
- 1 tablespoon sesame oil
- 1 tablespoon sunflower oil
- ½ teaspoon rosemary essential oil

Directions:

Place all the ingredients in a double boiler except the rosemary essential oil. Cook over low heat for 20 minutes to an hour.

To use: Apply on wet hair. Cover the hair with plastic cap for an hour. Rinse thoroughly with warm water.

Tip: If the hair is blond, add lemon essential oil instead of rosemary essential oil. 1 teaspoon of fresh lemon juice may also be added. The lemon will help highlight the blonde strands.

If the hair is dyed black, adding sage essential oil instead of rosemary essential oil is advised. Sage is known to darken the colors.

If the hair is red, add a teaspoon of beet or raspberry juice or oil.

If the hair is brown, add a teaspoon of coffee extract.

Hair Strengthening Hot Oil Treatment

Ingredients:

- 1 tablespoon jojoba oil
- 1 tablespoon castor oil
- 1 tablespoon sunflower or coconut oil
- 1 teaspoon sesame oil
- 5 drops carrot oil
- 5 drops rosemary oil

Directions:

Place the oils in a small bowl except for the carrot, rosemary and sesame oil. Heat the mixture in the microwave. Heating the oils in the double boiler can be an option, too. Heat the oil for 5 minutes in the microwave or for an hour, if using the double boiler.

Remove the oil from the fire and add the essential oils.

To use: Use the oil immediately while warm. Massage the oil to the scalp thoroughly. Cover the hair with plastic cap for an hour or wrap it with a hot towel. Rinse with warm water.

Hair Spray Recipe

Organic Citrus Hair Spray

Ingredients:

- 1 organic lemon
- 2 cups distilled or purified water
- 3 tablespoons clear grain alcohol or vodka
- 10 drops of essential oil

Directions:

Slice the lemon into wedges. Place it in a deep sauce pan. Add the water. Let it boil until the liquid is reduced to about 1 cup.

Strain the mixture using cheesecloth or a fine strainer. No lemon pulp should fall out with the liquid. Let the mixture cool down. Do not place the mixture in the fridge to cool. It may solidify the natural lemon oil.

Mix the essential oil and alcohol in a small bowl.

Add to the lemon mixture. Mix well. Place the mixture in a spray bottle and use.

Tip: If the hair is dark in color, substitute orange for the lemon. If the hair is red, substitute the lemon with grapefruit.

Chapter 6: Stocking and Storing your Essential Oil Products

Most essential carrier Oils and fragrance essential oils can last up to six months in the shelf. However, when these oils are used for hair and cosmetic products, the shelf life of the product may become lesser than that of the oil.

Some of the products would have a very short shelf life while others can last more than six months if stored carefully.

Below are some tips on how to stock or store your essential oil products.

1. If citrus fruits are added to the product, it can last for two to three months in the shelf. So, it is safe and practical to make it in bulk.

2. If fresh fruits or ingredients, such as avocado, banana and mangoes, are added to the hair product, the product can last for a week even if stored in the fridge.

Using the products beyond one week may cause adverse effects on the scalp and the skin.

*When using fruits or vegetables in the product, use only the organic fruits to make the product chemical free.

3. If yogurt is added to the hair product, it can last for three weeks in the fridge and one week on the shelf.

4. When the product contains eggs, make sure to use the product immediately. Though the product has an average shelf life of three days in the fridge, the risk of the existence of salmonella in the mixture gets higher every day.

5. If coconut milk is used, the product can last three weeks in the fridge, but can last only one week on the shelf.

   Expired coconut milk is still safe and actually beneficial when used on the hair. Just remove the curdled substances on top of the mixture. However, the product may emit an offensive smell which is similar to coconut vinegar. Adding chamomile oil to the mix can help neutralize the smell.

6. When storing products that need to be reheated or thawed before application, such as products with Shea butter or coconut oil, it is suggested to store them in small microwavable plastic sachets instead of big containers. It will be easier to reheat them.

Conclusion

Thank you again for downloading this book!

I hope this book was able to help you to make you appreciate how essential oils help make your hair strong, beautiful, shining and full of body. I also hope that you are encouraged to use healthy, chemical free and natural products on your hair.

The next step is to determine what type of hair you have now and try the all- natural products we recommended in this book. I hope that the products will have amazing results on your hair.

Also, when you find a product that suits your hair from this book, stick to using it for your daily hygiene or styling. Do not experiment with other commercial products for it may just damage your healthy hair again.

Finally, if you enjoyed this book, then I'd like to ask you for a favor, would you be kind enough to leave a review for this book on Amazon? It'd be greatly appreciated!

Thank you and good luck!